KIDNEY DISEASE COOKBOOK FOR STAGE 3

Low Sodium, Potassium and Phosphorus Recipes for Renal Diet

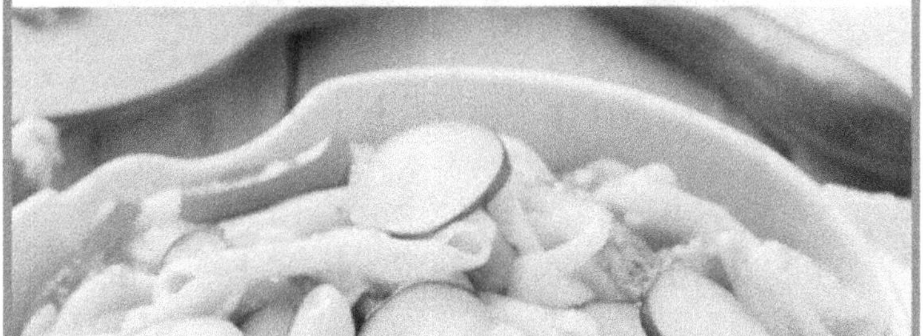

LISA T. JONES

TABLE OF CONTENT

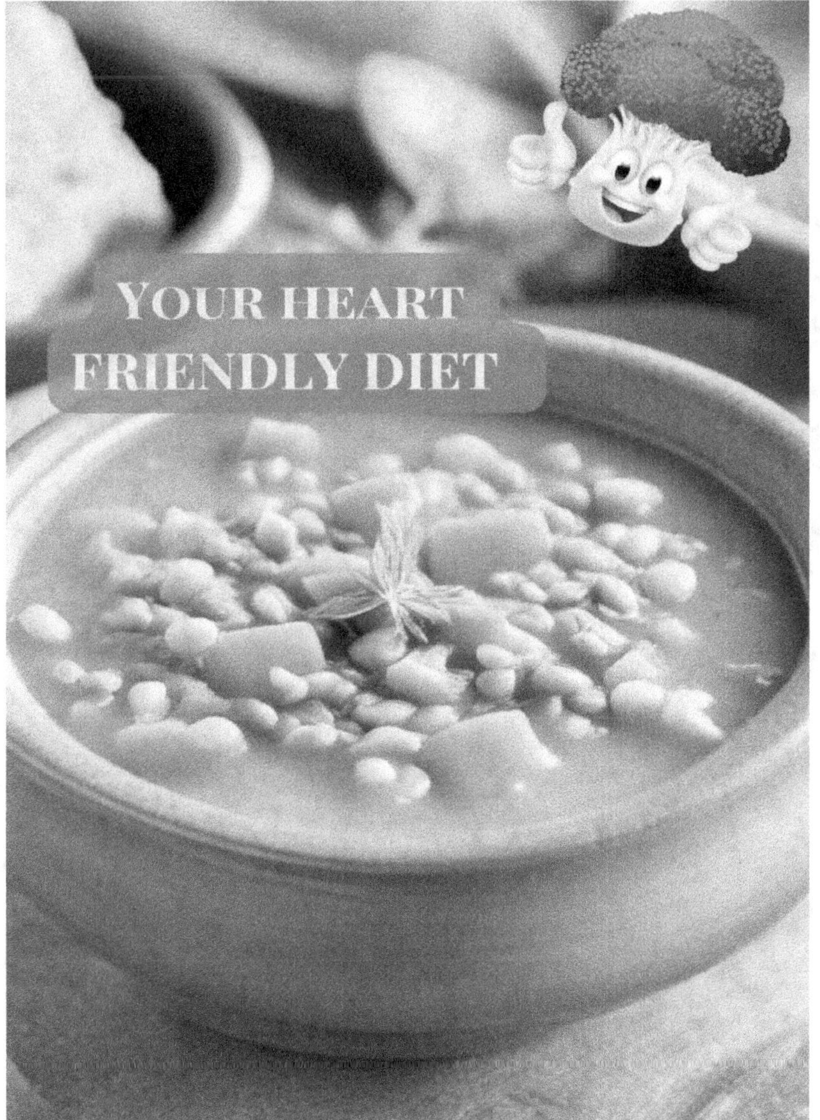

YOUR HEART
FRIENDLY DIET

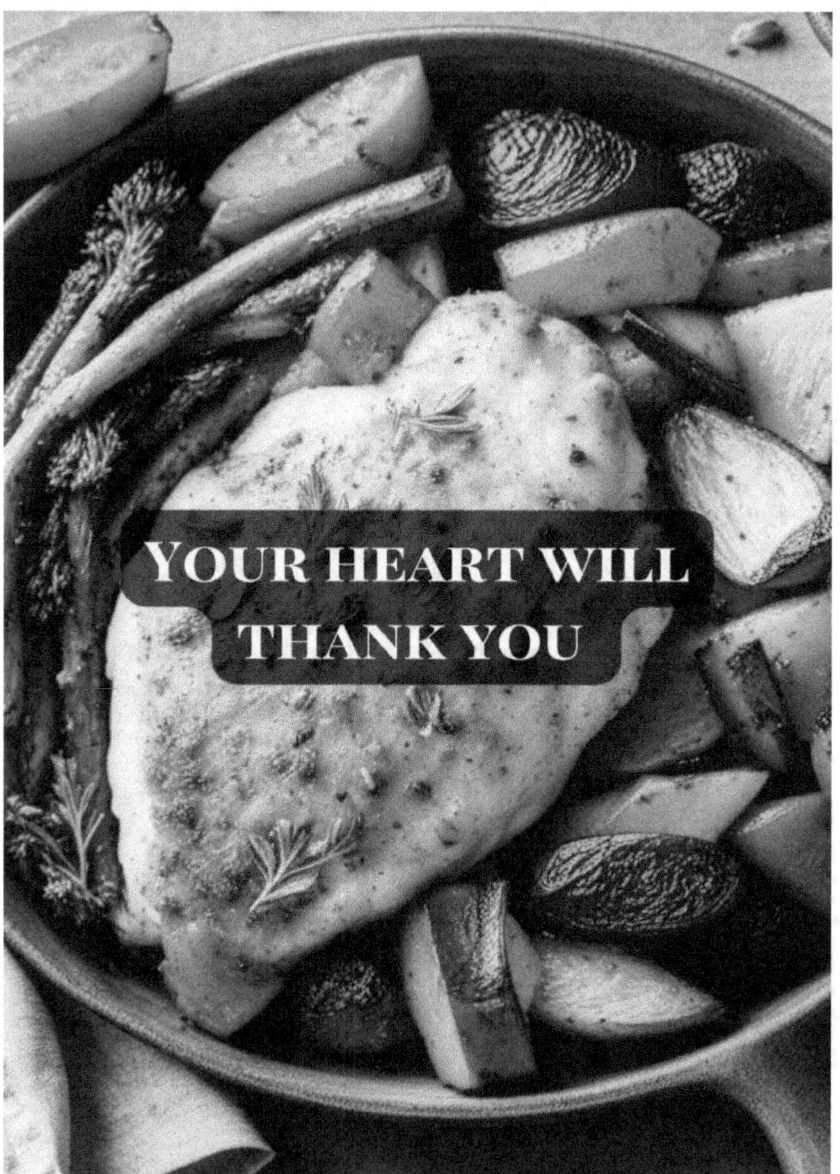
YOUR HEART WILL
THANK YOU

INTRODUCTION

Welcome to the Kidney Disease Cookbook for Stage 3, a friend in your journey to better health! If you've recently been handed a kidney disease diagnosis, I understand that it might feel like a curveball. It's natural to have worries and questions – after all, health matters are like uncharted territories.

But here's the thing: I'm not here to just talk about kidney disease; I'm here to show you how you can rewrite the story. We get it – change can be challenging, but remember, every superhero has their origin story. Consider this cookbook your starting point, your guide to embracing a healthier lifestyle that's filled with possibilities.

Guess what? You're not alone in this adventure. We're here to offer a helping hand, delicious recipes, and a sprinkle of hope. This cookbook isn't just about diets and numbers; it's about taking small steps that can lead to big wins. You have the power to manage your diagnosis and even reverse its effects with the right choices.

So let's cook up some tasty meals that not only nourish your body but also bring joy to your taste buds. We're on a mission to make this journey enjoyable, flavorful, and full of promise. Together, we'll create a recipe for success, health, and a brighter future.

Remember, every meal you prepare is a step toward a healthier you. It's time to embrace your inner superhero and embark on this exciting chapter. With a little bit of determination, a dash of creativity, and this cookbook as your trusty guide, you're well on your way to leading a healthy and vibrant life. Let's turn those challenges into victories, one delicious dish at a time!

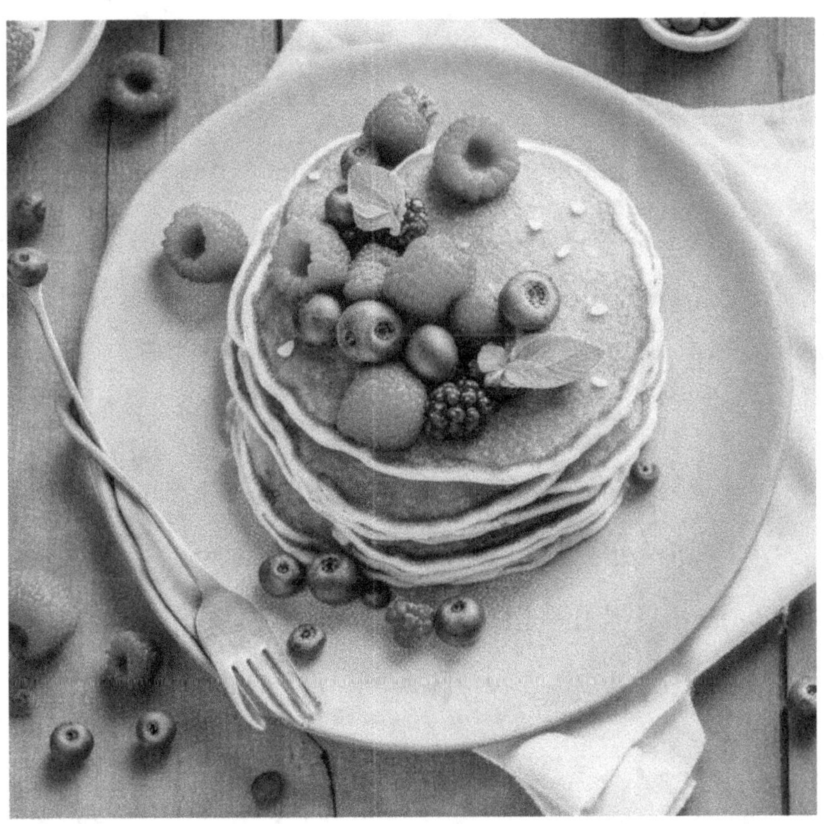

CHAPTER ONE

CORE BENEFITS OF FOLLOWING THE KIDNEY-FRIENDLY DIET

Just like you know how to take care of your daily needs, your body needs some special care too, especially if you have kidney disease. Let's explore how following a kidney disease diet can be a superhero move for seniors:

1. Super Kidney Strength:

Following a kidney disease diet gives your hardworking kidneys a break. Imagine them getting a spa day! They don't have to work as hard to clean out waste and fluids, which can help keep them stronger for longer.

2. Happy Heart:

When you stick to your kidney-friendly diet, you're not just helping your kidneys – you're also giving your heart a pat on the back. That's because a kidney diet often keeps salt and fluids in check, which can lower your blood pressure. A happy heart means a happier you!

3. Energy Boost:

Remember how you used to play with friends and have a good time? A kidney disease diet can help bring back some of that pep in your step. With the right nutrients, you'll have more energy to enjoy your hobbies, family time, and maybe even a dance or two.

4. Lowers blood pressure:

High blood pressure is a common problem for people with stage 3 kidney disease. Following a kidney-friendly diet can help to lower blood pressure, which can reduce your risk of heart disease, stroke, and other health problems.

5. Controls blood sugar levels:

Diabetes is another common problem for people with stage 3 kidney disease. Following a kidney-friendly diet can help to control blood sugar levels, which can reduce your risk of complications from diabetes.

6. Helps you lose weight:

Obesity is a risk factor for kidney disease. Losing weight can help to improve your kidney function and reduce your risk of developing other health problems. Following a kidney-friendly diet can help you to lose weight in a healthy way.

7. Strong Bones:

A kidney-friendly diet makes sure your bones stay sturdy. You won't need to worry about fractures or discomfort, allowing you to stay active and continue those lovely walks in the park.

8. Less Swelling, More Comfort:

Ever had those days when your feet and ankles swell up? A kidney disease diet can help control that. Imagine slipping into your favorite shoes without any hassle!

9. Smile on Your Face:

When you're feeling healthier, your mood often improves too. Imagine enjoying your favorite book or chatting with friends without any discomfort holding you back.

10. Keeps Medicine at Bay:

By eating right, you might not need as many medications to manage your health. Imagine having fewer pill bottles to deal with – that's a win!

11. Tasty Adventures:

Following a kidney disease diet doesn't mean boring meals. With the right recipes and a bit of creativity, you can enjoy delicious dishes that fit your diet and keep your taste buds happy.

12. More Quality Time:

Ultimately, a kidney disease diet helps you live your life to the fullest. Imagine being able to spend quality time with your loved ones, making cherished memories that will be talked about for generations.

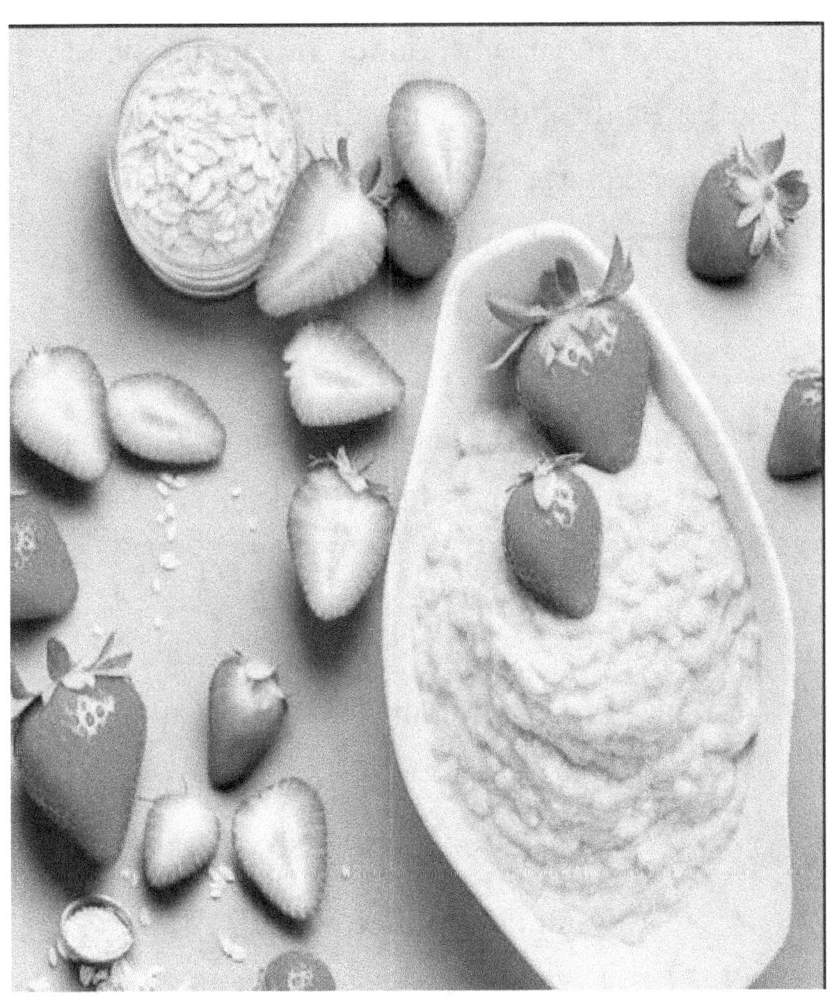

KIDNEY-FRIENDLY SHOPPING LIST

This kidney disease diet cookbook is designed to support kidney function, reduce stress on the kidney, and minimize the risk of further damage. For a kidney disease diet, it's important to manage protein, sodium, phosphorus, potassium, and fluid intake.

Here's a shopping list with kidney disease-friendly ingredients curated just for you:

PROTEIN

- Lean cuts of poultry (chicken, turkey)
- Fish (salmon, trout, cod)
- Eggs (in moderation)
- Low-fat dairy (milk, yogurt, cheese)

➢ Plant-based protein sources (tofu, tempeh, legumes)

CARBOHYDRATE

➢ Whole grains (whole wheat pasta, brown rice, quinoa)

➢ Fresh fruits (berries, apples, pears)

➢ Vegetables (leafy greens, bell peppers, zucchini)

HEALTHY FATS

➢ Avocado

➢ Nuts (almonds, walnuts)

➢ Seeds (flaxseeds, chia seeds)

➢ Olive oil

DAIRY AND ALTERNATIVES

➤ Low-fat or non-fat dairy products (milk, yogurt)

➤ Unsweetened almond milk or other low-phosphorus milk alternatives

BEVERAGES

➤ Water (stay well-hydrated, but follow doctor's recommendations on fluid intake)

➤ Herbal teas (avoid teas high in potassium)

LOW-POTASSIUM FRUITS

➤ Berries (strawberries, blueberries, raspberries)

➤ Apples

➤ Grapes

- ➢ Pineapple

LOW-POTASSIUM VEGETABLES

- ➢ Bell peppers

- ➢ Cabbage

- ➢ Cauliflower

- ➢ Lettuce

LOW-PHOSPHORUS CHOICES

- ➢ White rice

- ➢ White bread

- ➢ Non-cola sodas

- ➢ Non-dairy creamer

1. High-Potassium Foods:

- ➢ Bananas
- ➢ Oranges and orange juice
- ➢ Potatoes
- ➢ Tomatoes and tomato products (sauces, ketchup)
- ➢ Spinach
- ➢ Avocado

2. High-Phosphorus Foods:

- ➢ Dairy products (milk, yogurt, cheese)
- ➢ Nuts and nut butters
- ➢ Chocolate and cocoa
- ➢ Colas and dark sodas
- ➢ Processed meats (sausages, hot dogs)

3. High-Sodium Foods:

> ➤ Processed and canned foods

> ➤ Fast food and restaurant meals

> ➤ Packaged snacks (chips, pretzels)

> ➤ Deli meats and processed cheeses

> ➤ Condiments high in sodium (soy sauce, teriyaki sauce)

4. High-Protein Foods:

> ➤ Red meat (beef, lamb, pork)

> ➤ Organ meats (liver, kidneys)

> ➤ Shellfish

> ➤ High-protein energy bars and supplements

> ➤ Excessive intake of animal-based protein

5. High-Oxalate Foods:

➤ Spinach

➤ Rhubarb

➤ Beets

➤ Swiss chard

➤ Chocolate

6. Fluid-Restrictive Beverages:

➤ Carbonated beverages

➤ Energy drinks

➤ Excessive caffeinated drinks

➤ High-sugar beverages

7. High-Sugar Foods:

➤ Sugary desserts (cakes, cookies, pastries)

➤ Sugary cereals

➤ Sweetened beverages

➢ Candy and sugary snacks

8. Excess Salt and Salt-Containing Foods:

➢ High-sodium processed foods

➢ Canned soups and broths

➢ Salted snacks (chips, pretzels)

➢ High-sodium condiments (soy sauce, salad dressings)

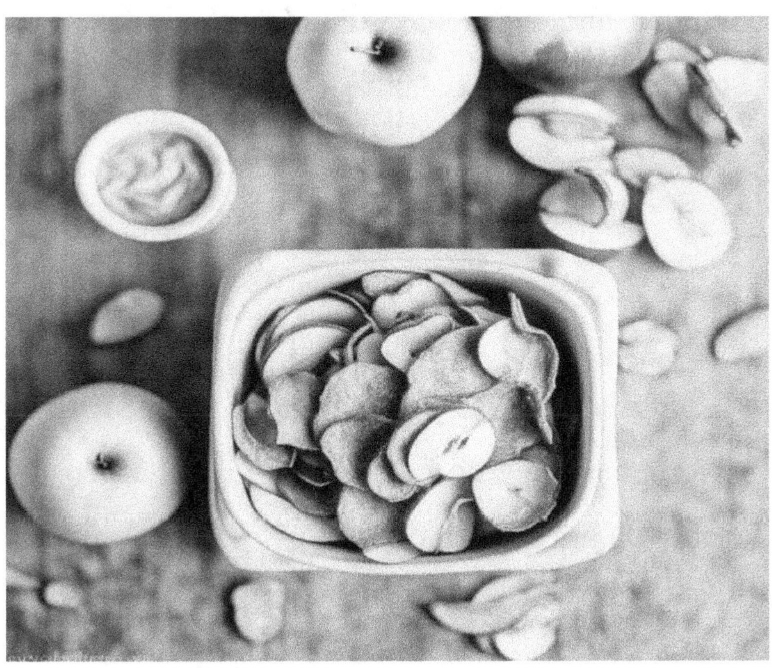

CHAPTER TWO

ALLERGEN INFORMATION

Whilst creating recipes suitable for most dietary restrictions, we understand the importance of safety and inclusivity. For these reasons, we'll clearly label potential COMMON allergens such as nuts, dairy, gluten, and more and suitable substitutes to achieve your tasty and healthy goal. Your well-being is our priority, and we want you to feel confident in your culinary choices.

However, it is important to check the label of all ingredients that you add to your meal to make sure they do not contain any allergens that you are sensitive to.

Ingredients	Allergens	Substitute
Tofu	Soy	Soy-free tofu/ Plant based protein
Cheese	Dairy	Lactose-free cheese
Wheat flour	Gluten	Gluten-free flour
Greek yogurt	Dairy	Dairy-free yogurt
Milk	Dairy	Dairy-free milk
Tzatziki sauce	Dairy (Yogurt)	Dairy-free yogurt
Egg	Egg	Egg substitute
Mayonnaise	Egg	Vegan mayonnaise

BREAKFAST

1. TOFU SCRAMBLE

This scramble is a good source of protein and fiber, and it's low in sodium and potassium. It's a vitamin and mineral rich food and an tasty source of iron and calcium.

Ingredients:

- 1 block extra-firm tofu, crumbled
- 1 tablespoon olive oil
- 1 onion, chopped
- 2 cloves garlic, minced
- 1 green bell pepper, chopped
- 1/2 teaspoon salt
- 1/4 teaspoon black pepper
- 1/4 teaspoon ground cumin

➢ 1/4 teaspoon paprika

Instructions:

➢ Over medium heat, heat the olive oil in a large wok.

➢ Add the tofu and cook until browned on all sides.

➢ Add the onion, garlic, bell pepper, salt, pepper, cumin, and paprika.

➢ Cook until the vegetables are softened, about 5 minutes.

Nutritional facts:

➢ Calories: 200

➢ Fat: 10 grams

➢ Saturated fat: 1 gram

➢ Carbohydrates: 10 grams

➢ Fiber: 5 grams

➢ Protein: 20 grams

2. COTTAGE CHEESE AND FRUIT BOWL

This cottage cheese and fruit bowl is a protein-packed and refreshing breakfast option.

Ingredients:

➢ ½ cup low-fat cottage cheese

➢ Sliced peaches or nectarines

➢ Chopped pistachios

➢ Drizzle of honey (optional)

Instructions:

➢ In a bowl, layer cottage cheese, sliced fruit, and chopped pistachios.

➢ Drizzle with honey if desired.

Nutritional Facts

➢ Calories: 250

➢ Protein: 15g

➢ Phosphorus: 200mg

➢ Potassium: 250mg

3. BERRY CHIA SEED PUDDING

Chia seeds are a great source of fiber and healthy fats, and berries are low in potassium, making this pudding a delicious and nutritious option.

Ingredients:

➢ 2 tablespoons chia seeds

- ➢ 1/2 cup unsweetened almond milk (or any low-phosphorus milk alternative)
- ➢ 1/4 teaspoon vanilla extract
- ➢ 1/2 cup mixed berries (such as strawberries, blueberries, raspberries)
- ➢ 1 teaspoon honey (optional, if desired)
- ➢ Chopped nuts (like almonds or walnuts), for garnish

Instructions:

- ➢ In a small bowl, mix chia seeds, almond milk, and vanilla extract. Stir well to combine.
- ➢ Cover the bowl and refrigerate for at least 2 hours or overnight, allowing the chia seeds to absorb the liquid and create a pudding-like texture.

➢ Once the chia pudding is set, give it a good stir to ensure the seeds are evenly distributed.

➢ Layer the chia pudding and mixed berries in a glass or jar, starting with a layer of pudding followed by a layer of berries.

➢ Repeat the layers until you've used up all the pudding and berries.

➢ If desired, drizzle a teaspoon of honey over the top for extra sweetness.

➢ Garnish with chopped nuts for added crunch and flavor.

Nutritional Facts

➢ Calories: 180

➢ Protein: 5g

➢ Phosphorus: 120mg

➢ Potassium: 150mg

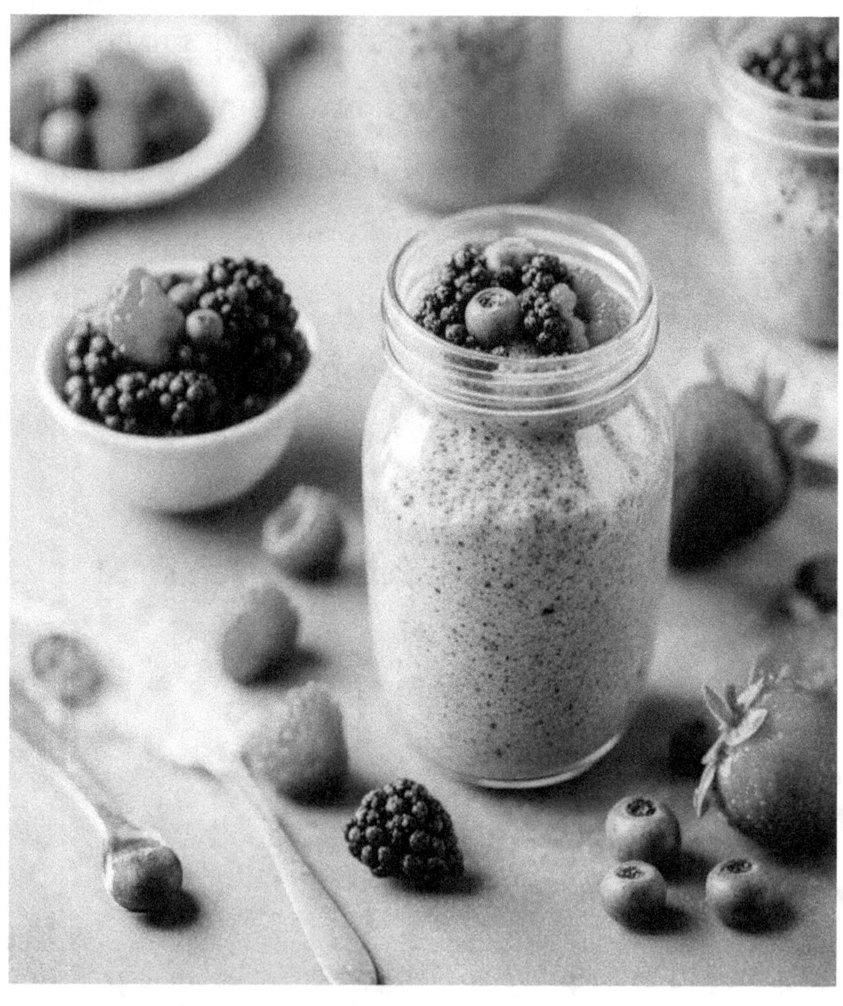

4. WHOLE GRAIN PANCAKES WITH BERRIES

These whole grain pancakes are a wholesome and kidney-friendly breakfast option, topped with antioxidant-rich berries.

Ingredients:

- ½ cup whole wheat flour
- ½ tsp baking powder
- 1 tbsp ground flaxseed
- ½ cup low-phosphorus milk or milk substitute
- Mixed berries for topping

Instructions:

- Mix flour, baking powder, and flaxseed.
- Stir in milk to create a batter.

➢ Cook pancakes on a nonstick skillet.

➢ Top with mixed berries.

Nutritional Facts

➢ Calories: 300

➢ Protein: 10g

➢ Phosphorus: 150mg

➢ Potassium: 200mg

5. OATMEAL WITH BERRIES

This oatmeal is a nutritious and filling option for breakfast. Oats provide fiber and berries add antioxidants. This dish is low in phosphorus and potassium.

Ingredients:

➢ ½ cup rolled oats

- ➢ 1 cup water or low-phosphorus milk

- ➢ ½ cup mixed berries (blueberries, strawberries)

Instructions:

- ➢ Cook oats in water or milk until soft.

- ➢ Top with mixed berries.

Nutritional Facts

- ➢ Calories: 250

- ➢ Protein: 8g

- ➢ Phosphorus: 150mg

- ➢ Potassium: 200mg

6. GREEK YOGURT PARFAIT

This parfait combines protein-rich Greek yogurt with fresh fruits and nuts for a satisfying and nutrient-dense breakfast.

Ingredients:

- ½ cup low-fat Greek yogurt
- ¼ cup mixed berries
- 1 tbsp chopped walnuts

Instructions:

- In a glass, layer Greek yogurt, berries, and walnuts.

Nutritional Facts

- Calories: 200
- Protein: 15g
- Phosphorus: 150mg

➢ Potassium: 200mg

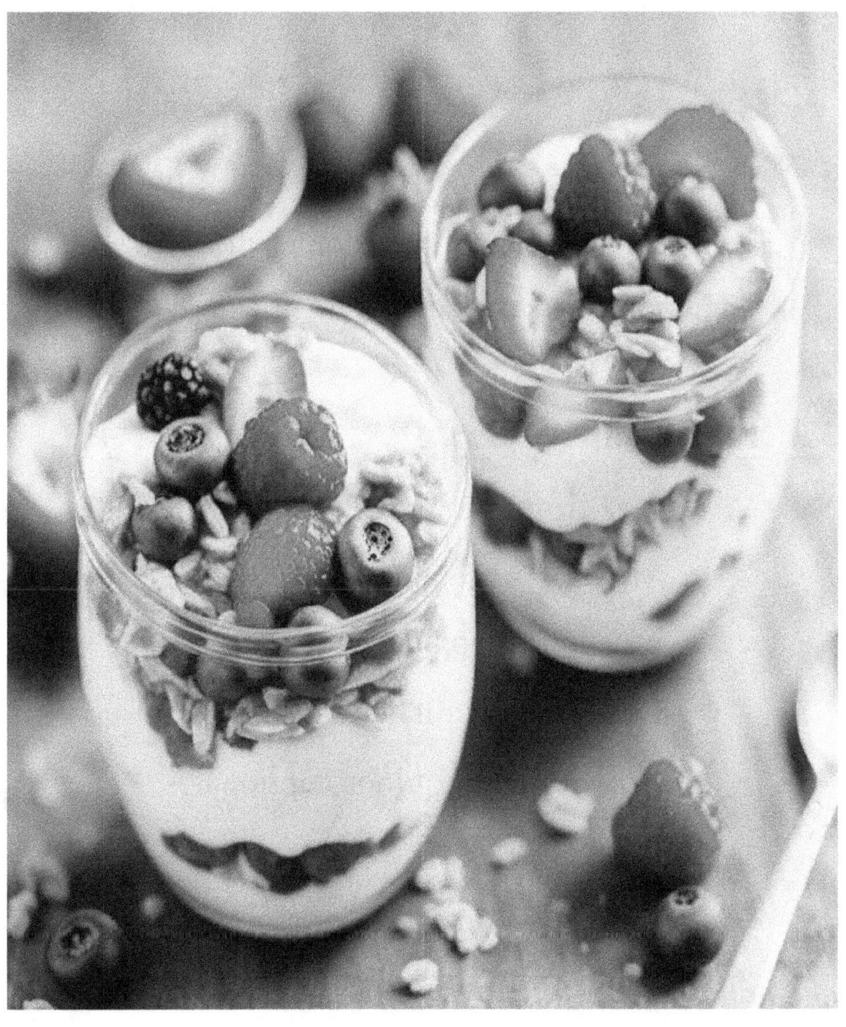

LUNCH

7. STIR-FRY TOFU WITH VEGETABLES

This stir-fry combines protein-rich tofu with a variety of colorful vegetables for a well-rounded lunch

Ingredients:

- ➢ 6 oz firm tofu, cubed
- ➢ Mixed vegetables (bell peppers, broccoli, snap peas)
- ➢ Low-sodium stir-fry sauce
- ➢ Brown rice or quinoa (optional)

Instructions:

- ➢ Sauté tofu and vegetables in a pan with stir-fry sauce.

> ➢ Serve over brown rice or quinoa if desired.

Nutritional Facts

> ➢ Calories: 300

> ➢ Protein: 15g

> ➢ Phosphorus: 200mg

> ➢ Potassium: 300mg

8. GRILLED PORTOBELLO MUSHROOMS

Grilled portobello mushrooms are a flavorful and satisfying main dish option, low in phosphorus and potassium.

Ingredients:

> ➢ 2 large portobello mushrooms

- ➤ Olive oil, balsamic vinegar
- ➤ Garlic, herbs

Instructions:

- ➤ Marinate mushrooms in olive oil, balsamic vinegar, garlic, and herbs.
- ➤ Grill until tender.

Nutritional Facts

- ➤ Calories: 150
- ➤ Protein: 5g
- ➤ Phosphorus: 100mg
- ➤ Potassium: 300mg

9. LEMON HERB BAKED SALMON

This baked salmon dish is rich in omega-3 fatty acids and is seasoned with herbs and lemon for a burst of flavor.

Ingredients:

- ➢ 6 oz salmon filet
- ➢ Lemon juice, herbs (dill, parsley)
- ➢ Olive oil

Instructions:

- ➢ Place salmon on a baking sheet, drizzle with olive oil and lemon juice.
- ➢ Sprinkle with herbs and bake until cooked through.

Nutritional Facts

- Calories: 300

- Protein: 30g

- Phosphorus: 250mg

- Potassium: 400mg

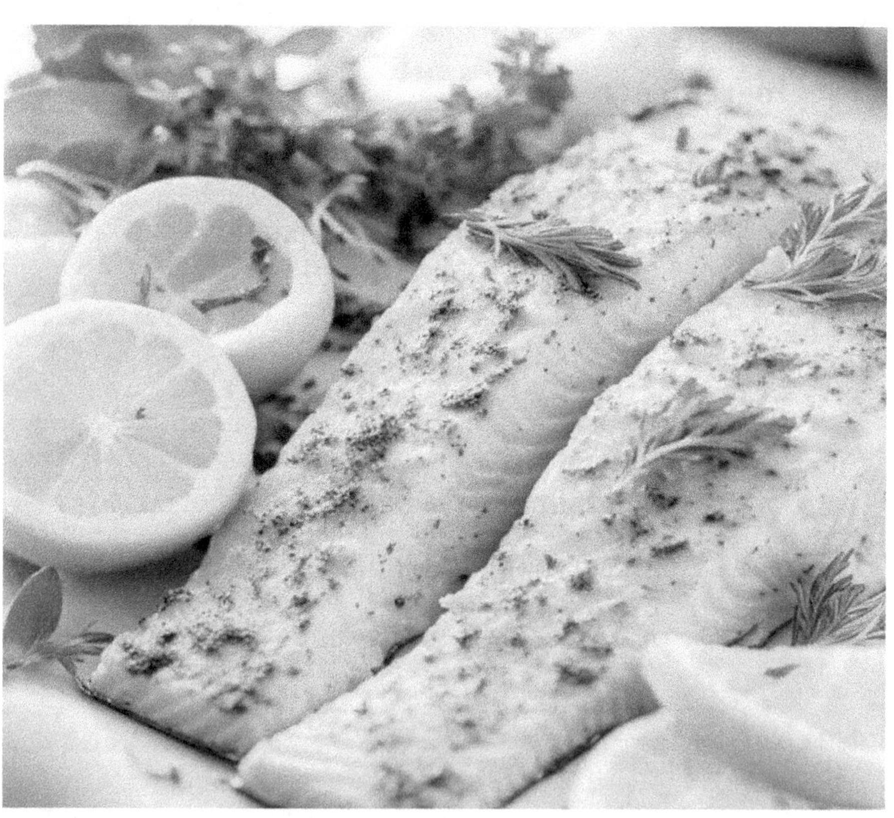

10.   TURKEY CHILI

This chili is a good source of protein and fiber, and it's low in sodium and potassium. It's also a good source of vitamins and minerals, including vitamin A, vitamin C, and potassium.

Ingredients:

- ➢ 1 pound ground turkey
- ➢ 1 onion, chopped
- ➢ 2 cloves garlic, minced
- ➢ 1 (15-ounce) can black beans, rinsed and drained
- ➢ 1 (15-ounce) can kidney beans, rinsed and drained
- ➢ 1 (14.5-ounce) can diced tomatoes, undrained
- ➢ 1 (15-ounce) can tomato sauce

- ➤ 1 teaspoon chili powder

- ➤ 1/2 teaspoon ground cumin

- ➤ 1/4 teaspoon salt

- ➤ 1/4 teaspoon black pepper

Instructions:

- ➤ In a large pot, brown the ground turkey over medium heat.

- ➤ Drain off any excess grease.

- ➤ Add garlic and onion and stir-fry it until it is tender

- ➤ Stir in the black beans, kidney beans, diced tomatoes, tomato sauce, chili powder, cumin, salt, and pepper.

- ➤ Bring to a boil, then reduce heat and simmer for 20 minutes, or until the flavors have blended.

Nutritional facts:

- ➤ Calories: 250
- ➤ Fat: 8 grams
- ➤ Saturated fat: 2 grams
- ➤ Carbohydrates: 25 grams
- ➤ Fiber: 6 grams
- ➤ Protein: 20 grams

11. TURKEY AND VEGETABLE WRAP

This wrap combines lean turkey, vegetables, and a whole wheat tortilla for a portable and balanced lunch option.

Ingredients:

- ➤ Whole wheat tortilla
- ➤ Sliced turkey breast

> Sliced vegetables (lettuce, tomato, cucumber)

> Hummus or mustard for spreading

Instructions:

> Lay out the tortilla and spread with hummus or mustard.

> Layer turkey and sliced vegetables.

> Roll up tightly to form a wrap.

Nutritional Facts

> Calories: 300

> Protein: 20g

> Phosphorus: 200mg

> Potassium: 300mg

12. EGGPLANT AND TOMATO RATATOUILLE

This flavorful ratatouille is a Mediterranean-inspired dish packed with vegetables and can be served warm or at room temperature.

Ingredients:

- ➤ 1 small eggplant, cubed
- ➤ Chopped tomatoes
- ➤ Sliced bell peppers
- ➤ Chopped onion
- ➤ Garlic, herbs (thyme, rosemary)

Instructions:

- ➤ Sauté onion and garlic until fragrant.
- ➤ Add eggplant, tomatoes, bell peppers, and herbs.
- ➤ Simmer until vegetables are tender.

Nutritional Facts

- ➢ Calories: 200

- ➢ Protein: 5g

- ➢ Phosphorus: 100mg

- ➢ Potassium: 300mg

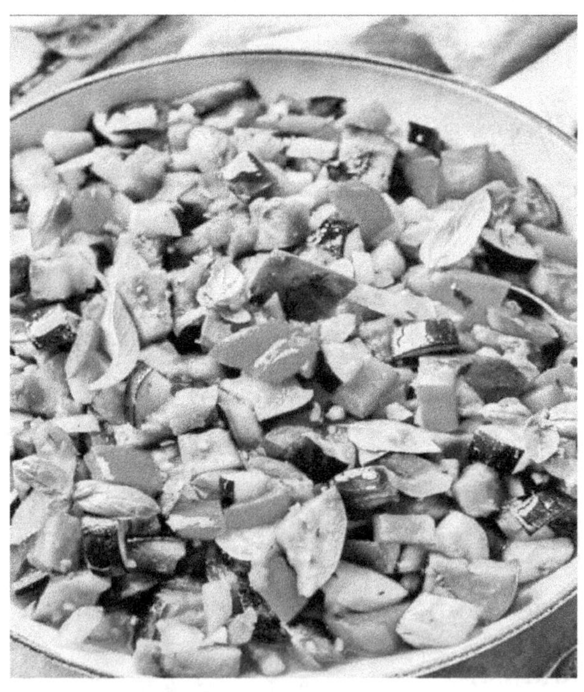

13. TUNA SALAD SANDWICH

This sandwich is a good source of protein and omega-3 fatty acids, and it's low in sodium and potassium. It's also a good source of vitamins and minerals, including vitamin D and vitamin B12.

Ingredients:

- 1 (12-ounce) can tuna, drained
- 1/2 cup mayonnaise
- 1/4 cup chopped celery
- 1/4 cup chopped onion
- 1 tablespoon lemon juice
- 1 teaspoon salt
- 1/4 teaspoon black pepper
- 2 slices whole-wheat bread

Instructions:

- ➤ In a bowl, combine the tuna, mayonnaise, celery, onion, lemon juice, salt, and pepper.
- ➤ Stir to combine.
- ➤ Spread the tuna salad on the bread.
- ➤ Serve immediately.

Nutritional facts:

- ➤ Calories: 250
- ➤ Fat: 10 grams
- ➤ Saturated fat: 1 gram
- ➤ Carbohydrates: 20 grams
- ➤ Fiber: 2 grams
- ➤ Protein: 20 grams

DINNER

14. SALMON WITH ROASTED VEGETABLES

This recipe is rich in vitamins, protein and omega-3 fatty acids. It's recipe also contains less amount of potassium and sodium.

Ingredients:

- 1 pound salmon filet, skin on
- 1 tablespoon olive oil
- 1 teaspoon salt
- 1/2 teaspoon black pepper
- 1 zucchini, sliced
- 1 yellow squash, sliced
- 1 red bell pepper, sliced
- 1/2 cup chopped onion

Instructions:

- Preheat the oven to 400°F (200°C)
- Brush the salmon filet with olive oil and season with salt and pepper.
- Place the salmon filet in a baking dish.
- Surround the salmon with the zucchini, yellow squash, red bell pepper, and onion.
- Bake for 20-25 minutes, or until the salmon is cooked through and the vegetables are tender.

Nutritional facts:

- Calories: 340
- Fat: 16 grams
- Saturated fat: 2 grams
- Carbohydrates: 10 grams
- Fiber: 4 grams

➢ Protein: 30 gram

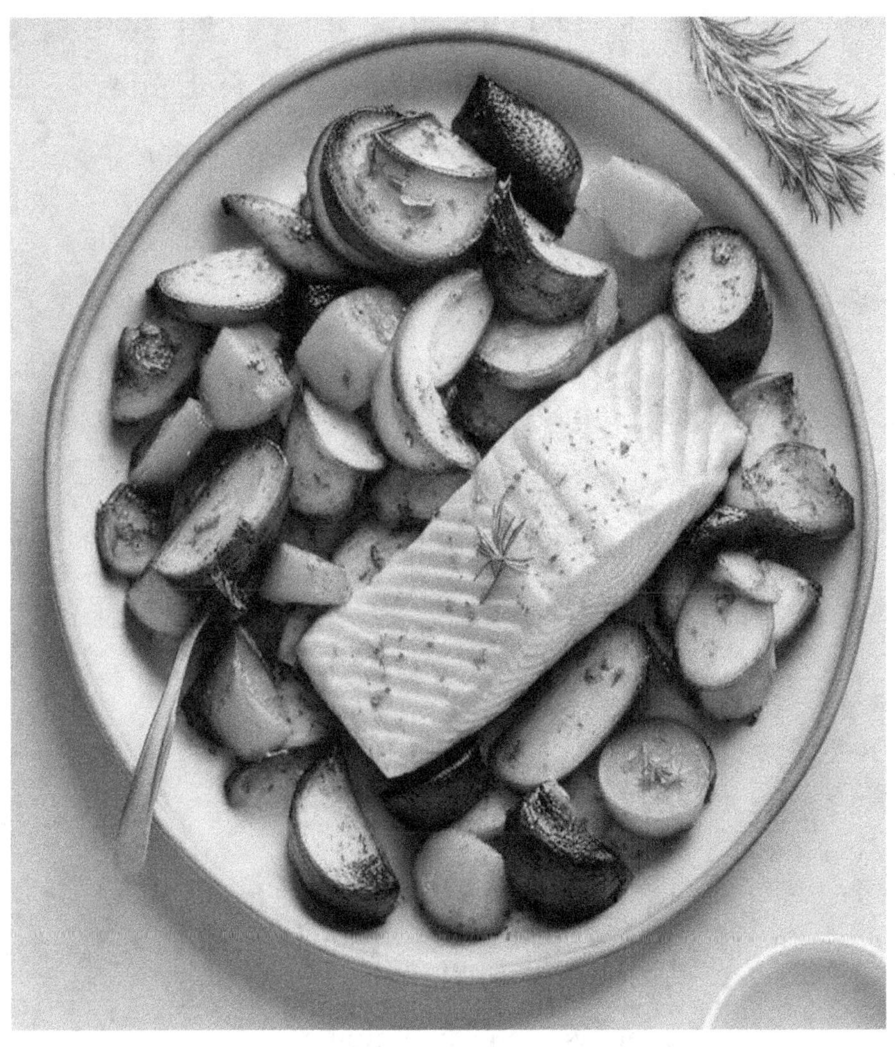

15. CHICKEN STIR-FRY

This stir-fry is a good source of protein and vegetables, and it's low in sodium and potassium. It's also a good source of vitamins and minerals, including vitamin A, vitamin C, and potassium.

Ingredients:

- 1 pound boneless, skinless chicken breasts, cut into bite-sized pieces
- 1 tablespoon olive oil
- 1 onion, chopped
- 2 carrots, chopped
- 1 red bell pepper, chopped
- 1 cup broccoli florets
- 1/2 cup snow peas
- 1/4 cup coconut aminos
- 1 tablespoon rice vinegar

- ➤ 1 teaspoon ground ginger

- ➤ 1/2 teaspoon garlic powder

- ➤ Salt and pepper to taste

Instructions:

- ➤ Heat the olive oil in a large skillet or wok over medium heat.

- ➤ Add the chicken and cook until browned on all sides.

- ➤ Add the onion, carrots, and bell pepper and cook until softened.

- ➤ Add the broccoli and snow peas and cook for 2-3 minutes, or until the vegetables are bright green.

- ➤ Stir in the coconut aminos, rice vinegar, ginger, garlic powder, salt, and pepper.

➢ Cook for 1-2 minutes, or until the sauce is heated through.

Nutritional facts:

➢ Calories: 280

➢ Fat: 12 grams

➢ Saturated fat: 3 grams

➢ Carbohydrates: 10 grams

➢ Fiber: 3 grams

➢ Protein: 30 grams

16.   CHICKEN KABOBS WITH TZATZIKI SAUCE

This dish is a good source of protein, and it's low in sodium and potassium. It's also a good source of vitamins and minerals, including vitamin A, vitamin C, and potassium.

Ingredients:

- 1 pound boneless, skinless chicken breasts, cubed (1-inch big)
- 1 tablespoon olive oil
- 1 teaspoon garlic powder
- 1/2 teaspoon salt
- 1/4 teaspoon black pepper
- 12 skewers, soaked in water for 30 minutes

➢ Tzatziki sauce (recipe below)

Instructions:

➢ In a large bowl, combine the chicken, olive oil, garlic powder, salt, and pepper.

➢ Thread the chicken onto the skewers.

➢ Grill the chicken kabobs over medium heat for 10-12 minutes, or until cooked through.

➢ Serve with tzatziki sauce.

Tzatziki sauce:

➢ 1 cup Greek yogurt

➢ 1 cucumber, peeled and diced

➢ 1/2 cup chopped dill

➢ 1/4 cup lemon juice

➢ 1/4 teaspoon salt

➢ 1/4 teaspoon black pepper

Instructions:

In a bowl, combine the Greek yogurt, cucumber, dill, lemon juice, salt, and pepper. Stir to combine.

Nutritional facts:

➢ Calories: 200

➢ Fat: 9 grams

➢ Saturated fat: 2 grams

➢ Carbohydrates: 6 grams

➢ Fiber: 2 grams

➢ Protein: 25 grams

17. VEGGIE BURGER

This burger is a good source of protein and fiber, and it's low in sodium and potassium. It's also a recipe rich in minerals and vitamins which includes calcium and iron.

Ingredients:

- 1 (15-ounce) can black beans, rinsed and drained
- 1 (15-ounce) can kidney beans, rinsed and drained
- 1/2 cup oats
- 1/2 cup chopped onion
- 1/4 cup chopped red bell pepper
- 1/4 cup chopped celery
- 1 egg, beaten
- 1 tablespoon olive oil
- 1 teaspoon garlic powder

- 1/2 teaspoon salt

- 1/4 teaspoon black pepper

Instructions:

- In a food processor, combine the black beans, kidney beans, oats, onion, bell pepper, celery, egg, olive oil, garlic powder, salt, and pepper.

- Process until smooth.

- Form the mixture into patties.

- Heat a large skillet over medium heat.

- Cook the patties for 5-7 minutes per side, or until cooked through.

Nutritional facts:

- Calories: 200

- Fat: 8 grams

- Saturated fat: 1 gram

➢ Carbohydrates: 20 grams

➢ Fiber: 6 grams

➢ Protein: 12 grams

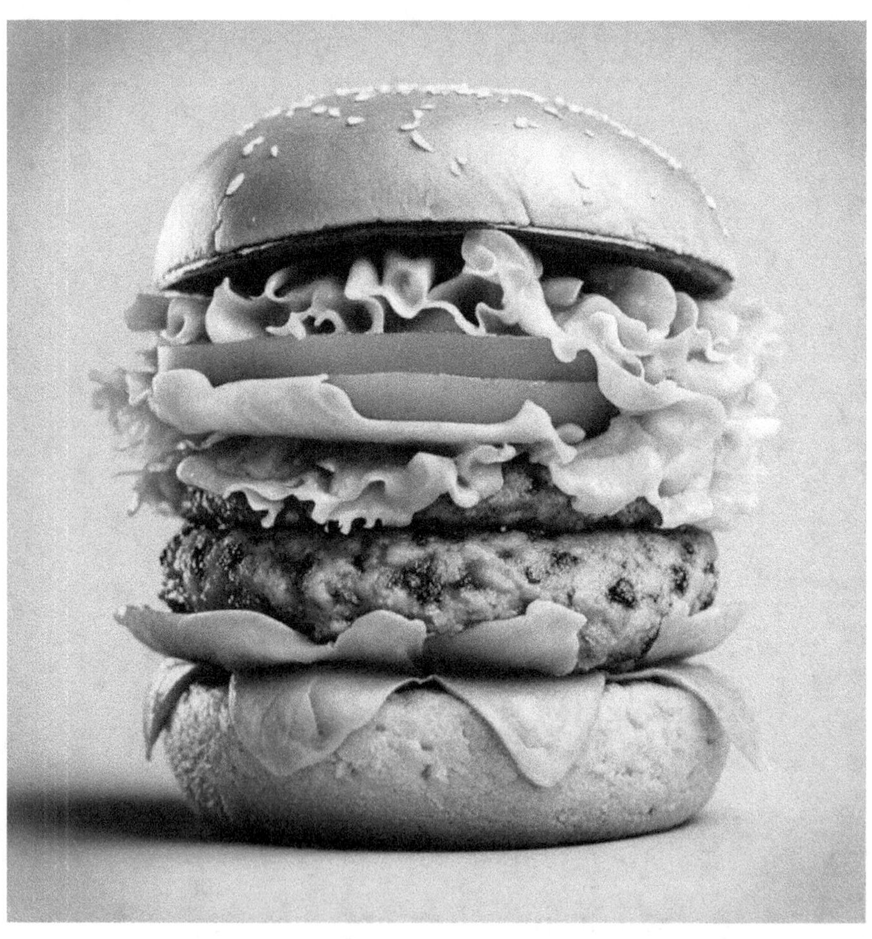

18. HERB-GRILLED CHICKEN WITH BROWN RICE AND STEAMED BROCCOLI

This meal is low in sodium, phosphorus, and potassium, making it a nutritious choice for kidney health.

Ingredients:

- 2 boneless, skinless chicken breasts
- 1 teaspoon dried thyme
- 1 teaspoon dried rosemary
- 1/2 teaspoon garlic powder
- Salt and black pepper, to taste
- 1 cup cooked brown rice
- 2 cups broccoli florets
- Lemon wedges, for garnish

Instructions:

- ➤ Preheat the grill or grill pan over medium heat.

- ➤ In a small bowl, mix the dried thyme, dried rosemary, garlic powder, salt, and black pepper.

- ➤ Lightly coat the chicken breasts with cooking spray or olive oil.

- ➤ Sprinkle the herb mixture over both sides of the chicken breasts.

- ➤ Grill the chicken breasts for about 4-5 minutes on each side, or until they are cooked through and have nice grill marks.

- ➤ While the chicken is grilling, steam the broccoli florets for about 3-4 minutes, or until they are tender but still vibrant green.

- ➤ Serve the herb-grilled chicken over a bed of cooked brown rice, with the steamed broccoli on the side.

- ➤ Garnish with lemon wedges for a burst of freshness.

Nutritional Facts:

- ➤ Calories: 350

- ➤ Protein: 30g

- ➤ Phosphorus: 220mg

- ➤ Potassium: 300mg

SNACKS

19.   RICE CAKES WITH HUMMUS

Rice cakes with hummus make a satisfying and kidney-friendly snack option.

Ingredients:

- ➢ Rice cakes
- ➢ Low-sodium hummus
- ➢ Sliced cucumbers or bell peppers

Instructions:

- ➢ Spread hummus on rice cakes.
- ➢ Top with sliced vegetables.

Nutritional Facts

- ➢ Calories: 100

- ➢ Protein: 3g

- ➢ Phosphorus: 50mg

- ➢ Potassium: 100mg

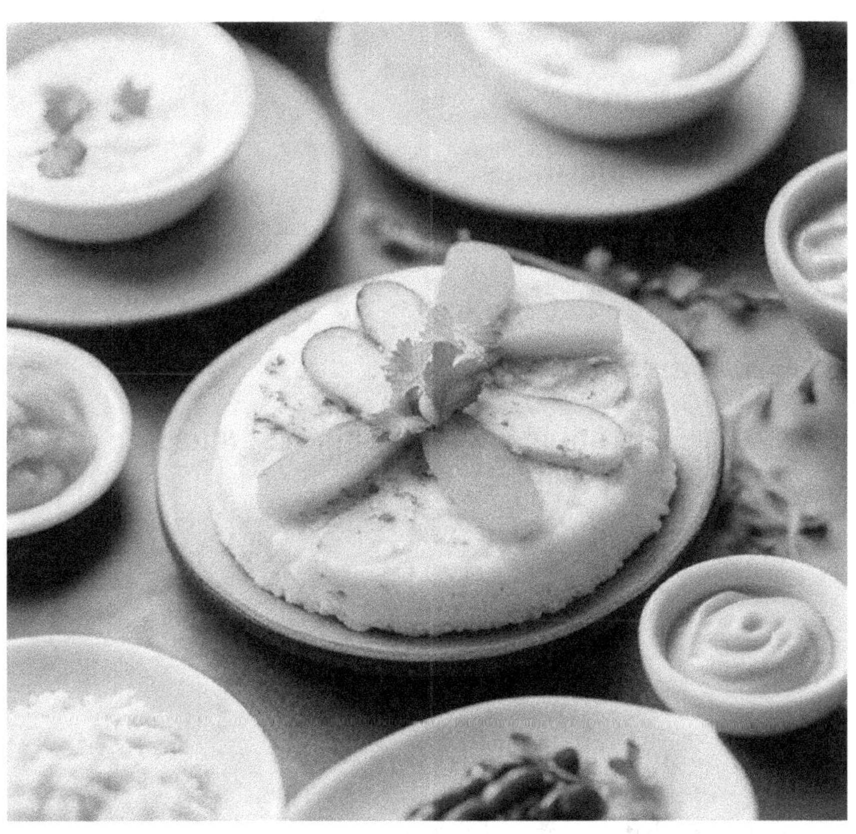

20. APPLE SLICES WITH ALMOND BUTTER

This simple snack combines the natural sweetness of apple slices with the protein and healthy fats of almond butter.

Ingredients:

- ➤ Apple slices
- ➤ Almond butter (unsalted)

Instructions:

- ➤ Dip apple slices in almond butter.

Nutritional Facts

- ➤ Calories: 150
- ➤ Protein: 3g
- ➤ Phosphorus: 100mg
- ➤ Potassium: 150mg

21. RICE CAKE WITH AVOCADO AND TOMATO

This snack pairs the creaminess of avocado with the freshness of tomato on a low-sodium rice cake.

Ingredients:

- ➤ Rice cake
- ➤ ¼ avocado, sliced
- ➤ Sliced tomato
- ➤ Dash of lemon juice

Instructions:

- ➤ Top rice cake with avocado and tomato slices.
- ➤ Drizzle with lemon juice.

Nutritional Facts

- ➤ Calories: 120

- ➣ Protein: 2g

- ➣ Phosphorus: 50mg

- ➣ Potassium: 150mg

22. ROASTED CHICKPEAS

Roasted chickpeas are a crunchy and protein-rich snack option that can be customized with different seasonings.

Ingredients:

- ➣ 1 can (15 oz) chickpeas, rinsed and drained

- ➣ Olive oil

- ➣ Seasonings (paprika, cumin, garlic powder)

Instructions:

- ➤ Toss chickpeas with olive oil and desired seasonings.
- ➤ Roast in the oven until crispy.

Nutritional Facts

- ➤ Calories: 150
- ➤ Protein: 6g
- ➤ Phosphorus: 100mg
- ➤ Potassium: 200mg

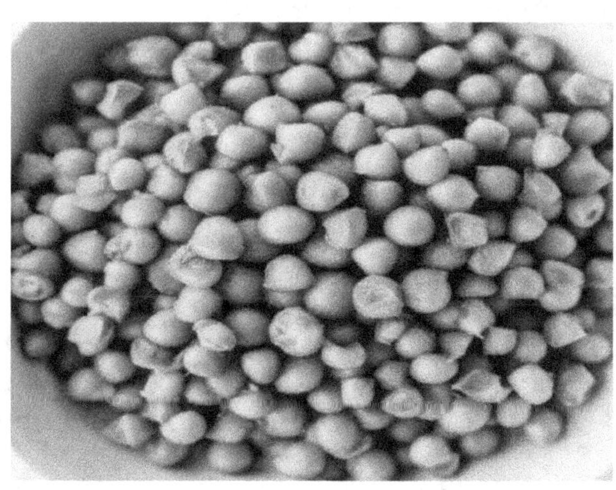

SOUPS AND SALADS

23. CREAMY BROCCOLI SOUP

This creamy broccoli soup is low in phosphorus and potassium while providing a good amount of vitamins and fiber.

Ingredients:

- ➤ 2 cups broccoli florets
- ➤ 1 onion, chopped
- ➤ 2 cups low-sodium vegetable broth
- ➤ ½ cup low-fat milk or milk substitute

Instructions:

- ➤ Sauté onion and broccoli in a pot until softened.

> Add vegetable broth and simmer until broccoli is tender.

> Blend until smooth, then stir in milk.

Nutritional Facts

> Calories: 150

> Protein: 5g

> Phosphorus: 150mg

> Potassium: 250mg

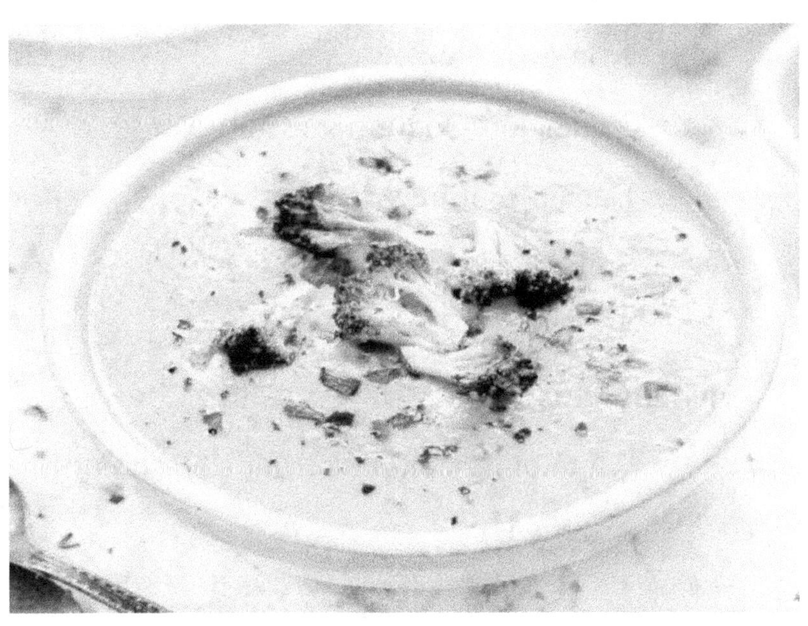

24. BUTTERNUT SQUASH SOUP

Creamy and flavorful, butternut squash soup is rich in vitamins and fiber, with a low phosphorus and potassium content.

Ingredients:

- ➢ 1 small butternut squash, peeled and cubed
- ➢ 1 onion, chopped
- ➢ 2 cups low-sodium vegetable broth
- ➢ Dash of nutmeg
- ➢ Salt and pepper to taste

Instructions:

- ➢ Sauté onion and butternut squash until softened.

➢ Add vegetable broth and simmer until squash is tender.

➢ Blend until smooth, adding nutmeg, salt, and pepper.

Nutritional Facts

➢ Calories: 150

➢ Protein: 2g

➢ Phosphorus: 100mg

➢ Potassium: 300mg

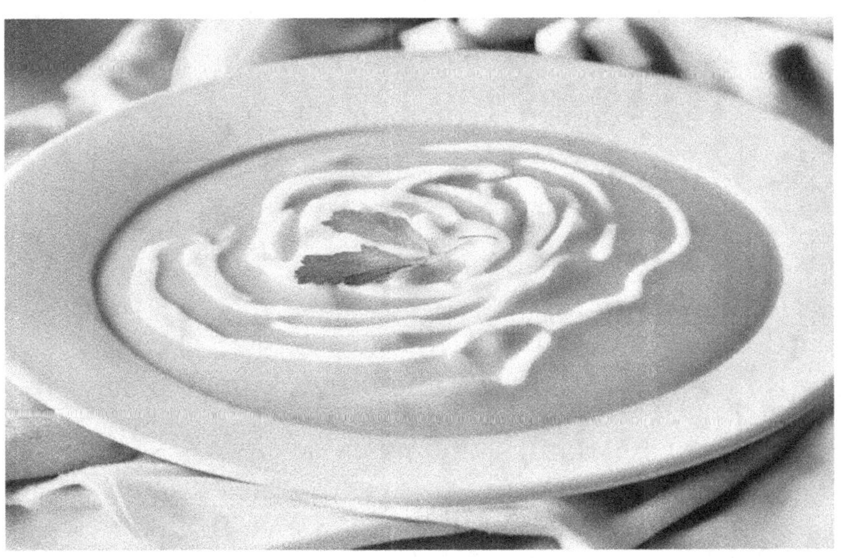

25.   MINESTRONE SOUP

Minestrone soup is a hearty and fiber-packed option that's versatile and customizable. Use low-phosphorus vegetables.

Ingredients:

- ➤ 1 cup low-sodium vegetable broth
- ➤ ½ cup cooked kidney beans (canned, drained, rinsed)
- ➤ Chopped low-phosphorus vegetables (zucchini, carrots, lettuce)
- ➤ ½ cup cooked whole wheat pasta
- ➤ Italian herbs and spices

Instructions:

- ➤ In a pot, combine broth, kidney beans, vegetables, and pasta.
- ➤ Season with Italian herbs and spices.

➢ Simmer until vegetables are tender.

Nutritional Facts

- ➢ Calories: 200
- ➢ Protein: 8g
- ➢ Phosphorus: 150mg
- ➢ Potassium: 300mg

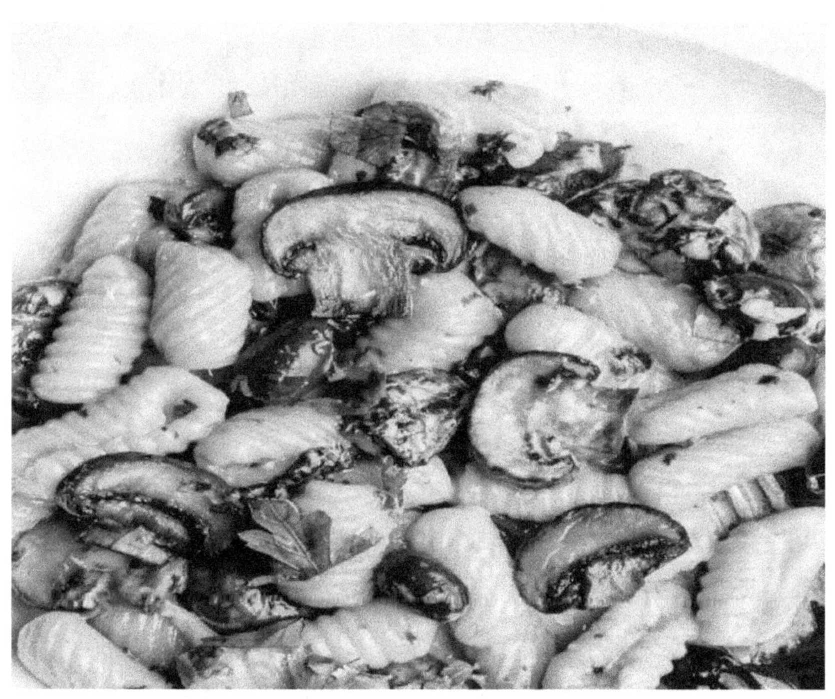

26.   CHICKEN SOUP

This soup is a good source of protein and fluids, and it's low in sodium and potassium. It's also a good source of vitamins and minerals, including vitamin A, vitamin C, and potassium.

Ingredients:

- 1 pound boneless, skinless chicken breasts, cut into bite-sized pieces
- 6 cups chicken broth
- 1 onion, chopped
- 2 carrots, chopped
- 2 celery stalks, chopped
- 1 bay leaf
- 1 teaspoon dried thyme
- 1/2 teaspoon salt
- 1/4 teaspoon black pepper

Instructions:

- ➤ In a large pot, combine the chicken, chicken broth, onion, carrots, celery, bay leaf, thyme, salt, and pepper. Leave the mixture to boil, turn to low heat and leave to cook for 20 minutes, or until the chicken is thoroughly cooked.
- ➤ Shred the thoroughly cooked chicken.
- ➤ Return the shredded chicken to the pot and stir to combine.

Nutritional facts:

- ➤ Calories: 200
- ➤ Fat: 4 grams
- ➤ Saturated fat: 1 gram
- ➤ Carbohydrates: 10 grams
- ➤ Fiber: 2 grams

➤ Protein: 25 grams

27. LENTIL SOUP

This soup is a good source of protein and fiber, and it's low in sodium and potassium. It's also a good source of vitamins and minerals, including folate, potassium, and magnesium.

Ingredients:

➤ 1 cup lentils, rinsed and drained

➤ 1 onion, chopped

➤ 2 carrots, chopped

➤ 2 celery stalks, chopped

➤ 4 cloves garlic, minced

➤ 6 cups vegetable broth

➤ 1 teaspoon dried thyme

- ➢ 1/2 teaspoon dried oregano

- ➢ 1/4 teaspoon ground black pepper

- ➢ Salt to taste

Instructions:

- ➢ In a large pot, combine the lentils, onion, carrots, celery, garlic, vegetable broth, thyme, oregano, and black pepper.

- ➢ Boil the combined ingredients. After, reduce heat and leave to simmer for 30 minutes, or until the lentils are soft.

- ➢ Season with salt to taste.

Nutritional facts:

- ➢ Calories: 230

- ➢ Fat: 4 grams

- ➢ Saturated fat: 1 gram

- ➤ Carbohydrates: 34 grams

- ➤ Fiber: 10 grams

- ➤ Protein: 12 grams

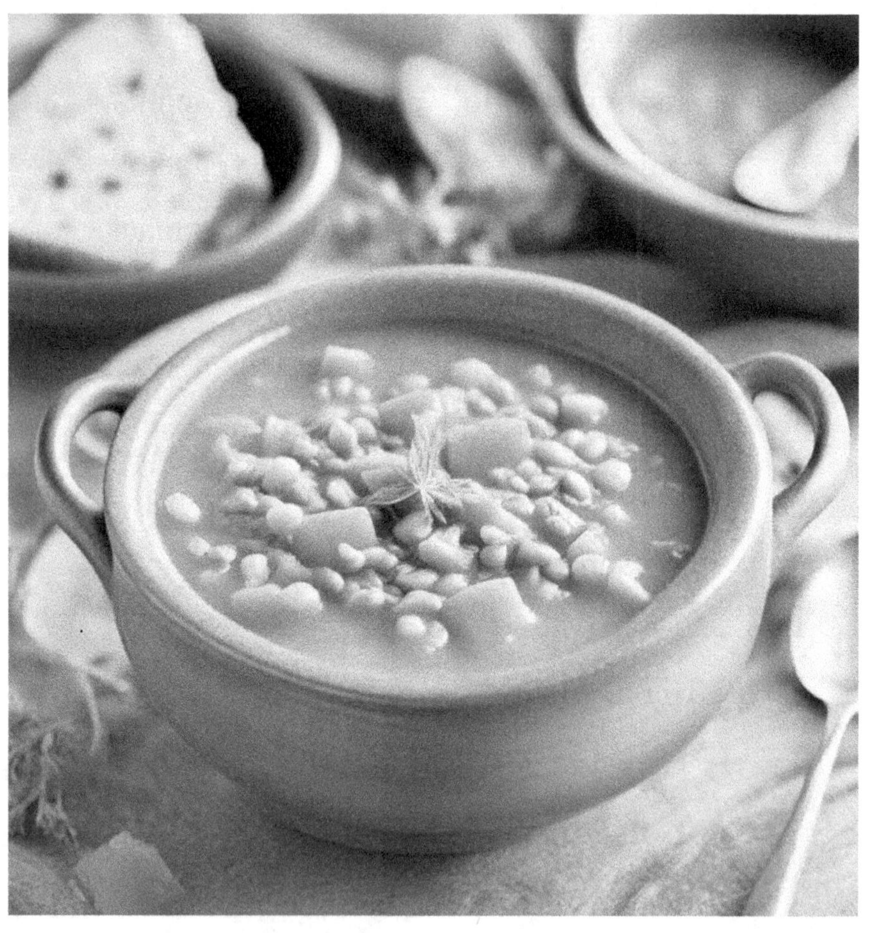

28. BLACK BEAN SOUP

This soup is a good source of protein, fiber, and iron, and it's low in sodium and potassium. It's contains folate, magnesium, and potassium which makes it a vitamin and mineral rich food.

Ingredients:

- 1 tablespoon olive oil
- 1 onion, chopped
- 2 cloves garlic, minced
- 1 (15-ounce) can black beans, rinsed and drained
- 1 (15-ounce) can kidney beans, rinsed and drained
- 1 (14.5-ounce) can diced tomatoes, undrained
- 1 (15-ounce) can tomato sauce

- ➤ 1 teaspoon chili powder

- ➤ 1/2 teaspoon ground cumin

- ➤ 1/4 teaspoon salt

- ➤ 1/4 teaspoon black pepper

Instructions:

- ➤ Over medium heat, heat the olive oil in a large pot.

- ➤ Add garlic and onion and cook until it's tender

- ➤ Stir in the black beans, kidney beans, diced tomatoes, tomato sauce, chili powder, cumin, salt, and pepper.

- ➤ Bring to a boil, then reduce heat and simmer for 20 minutes, or until the flavors have blended.

Nutritional facts:

- ➢ Calories: 220
- ➢ Fat: 5 grams
- ➢ Saturated fat: 1 gram
- ➢ Carbohydrates: 28 grams
- ➢ Fiber: 10 grams
- ➢ Protein: 14 grams

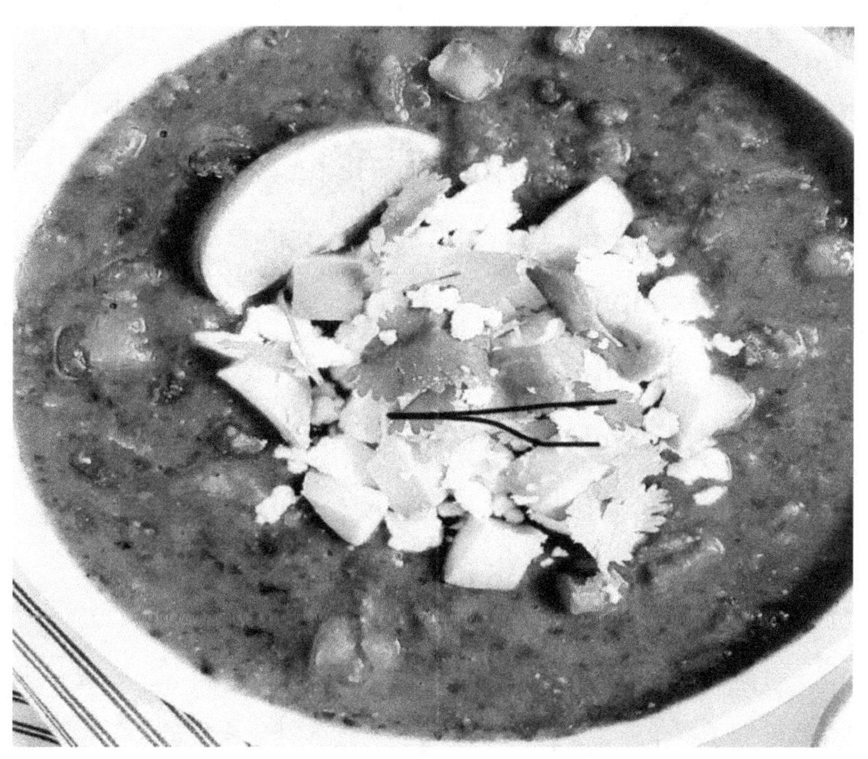

29. VEGETABLE SALAD

This salad is a good source of vitamins, minerals, and fiber, and it's low in sodium and potassium. It's a perfect way to reach your daily requirements of vegetables and fruits

Ingredients:

- Any combination of your favorite vegetables, such as lettuce, tomatoes, carrots, cucumbers, peppers, and onions
- 1 tablespoon olive oil
- 1/2 teaspoon salt
- 1/4 teaspoon black pepper
- 1/4 teaspoon dried oregano
- 1/4 teaspoon dried basil

Instructions:

- ➢ Wash and chop the vegetables.
- ➢ In a large bowl, combine the vegetables, olive oil, salt, pepper, oregano, and basil.
- ➢ Toss to coat.

Nutritional facts:

- ➢ Calories: 100
- ➢ Fat: 10 grams
- ➢ Saturated fat: 1 gram
- ➢ Carbohydrates: 10 grams
- ➢ Fiber: 5 grams
- ➢ Protein: 2 grams

30.   **GRILLED CHICKEN SALAD**

This salad is a balanced and kidney-friendly lunch option. The combination of grilled chicken, fresh vegetables, and low-sodium dressing provides protein and vitamins without excessive phosphorus or potassium.

Ingredients:

➤ 4 oz grilled chicken breast

➤ Mixed salad greens

➤ Cucumber, tomato, red onion

➤ Balsamic vinaigrette (low-sodium)

Instructions:

➤ Arrange salad greens, vegetables, and grilled chicken on a plate.

➤ Drizzle with balsamic vinaigrette.

Nutritional Facts

➢ Calories: 300

➢ Protein: 30g

➢ Phosphorus: 250mg

➢ Potassium: 350mg

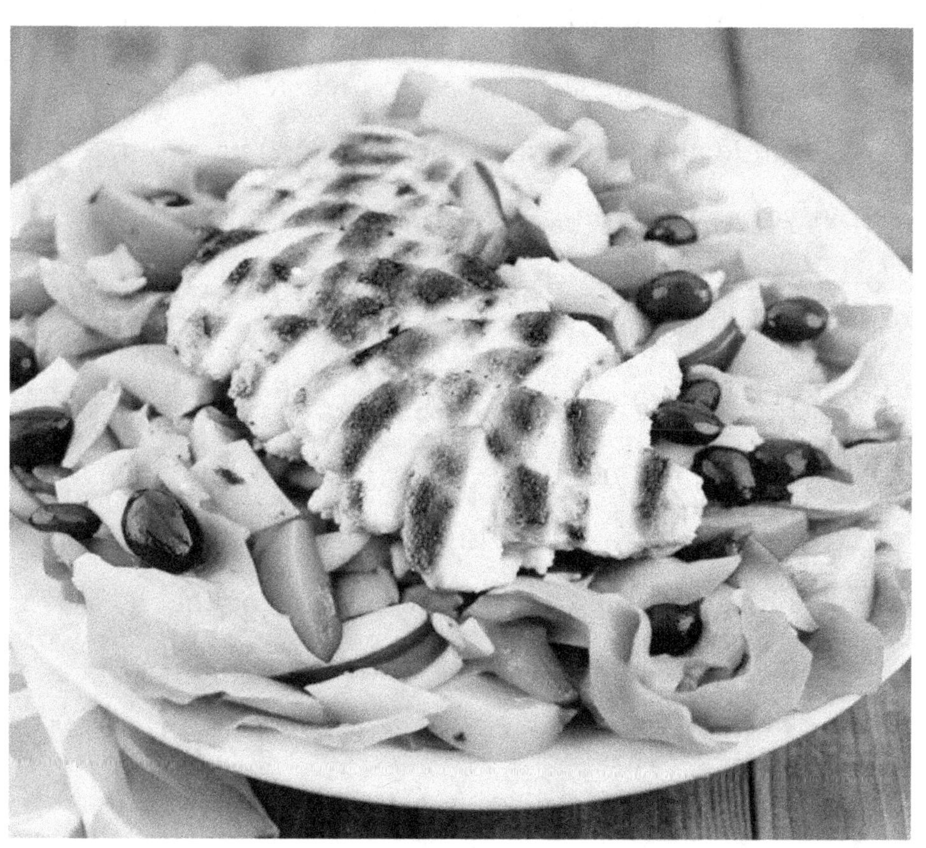

CONCLUSION

As we reach the final pages of the Kidney Disease Cookbook For Stage 3, we want to extend our heartfelt gratitude for joining us on this nourishing journey. From the first recipe to the last, we've aimed to create a guide that's not just about food, but about your well-being, your strength, and your resilience.

Embracing a kidney disease diet is a powerful choice – one that empowers you to take charge of your health and live life to the fullest. Remember, this isn't just a cookbook; it's a testament to your determination, your commitment to self-care, and your unwavering spirit.

As you savor each meal and savor each moment, know that you're making a positive impact on your life. Every ingredient you choose, every recipe you create, and every step you take toward a healthier lifestyle is a step toward a brighter future.

So, here's to you – the hero of your story. You've shown strength in the face of challenges, and you've discovered that delicious and nutritious can indeed go hand in hand. As you continue on this path, know that you're never alone. We're here to support you, cheer you on, and celebrate your successes.

Now, as you close this cookbook and step into the world with newfound knowledge and recipes in hand, remember this: your health matters, your journey matters, and you matter. Embrace this diet, adapt it to your needs, and watch as your life transforms.

You're the artist that wields the brush that paints on the canvas of your body, the outcome of that work of art depends on you. With each mindful choice, you're painting a masterpiece of health, happiness, and vitality. So, go ahead – take the first bite, savor the flavors, and let this journey be a reminder that you have the power to create the life you deserve.

Here's to your health, here's to your future, and here's to you. You've got this – and we believe in you every step of the way. Let the Kidney Disease Cookbook for Stage 3 be your guide, your companion, and your inspiration to live a life that's vibrant, nourished, and truly extraordinary. Your journey is only beginning, and the best is yet to come!

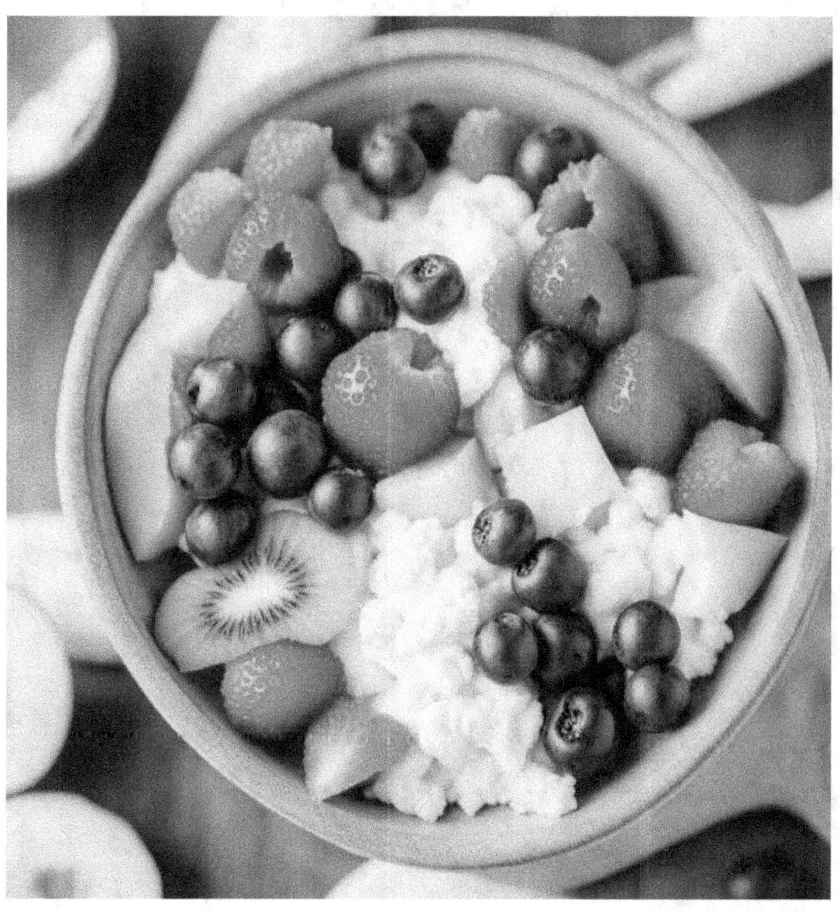

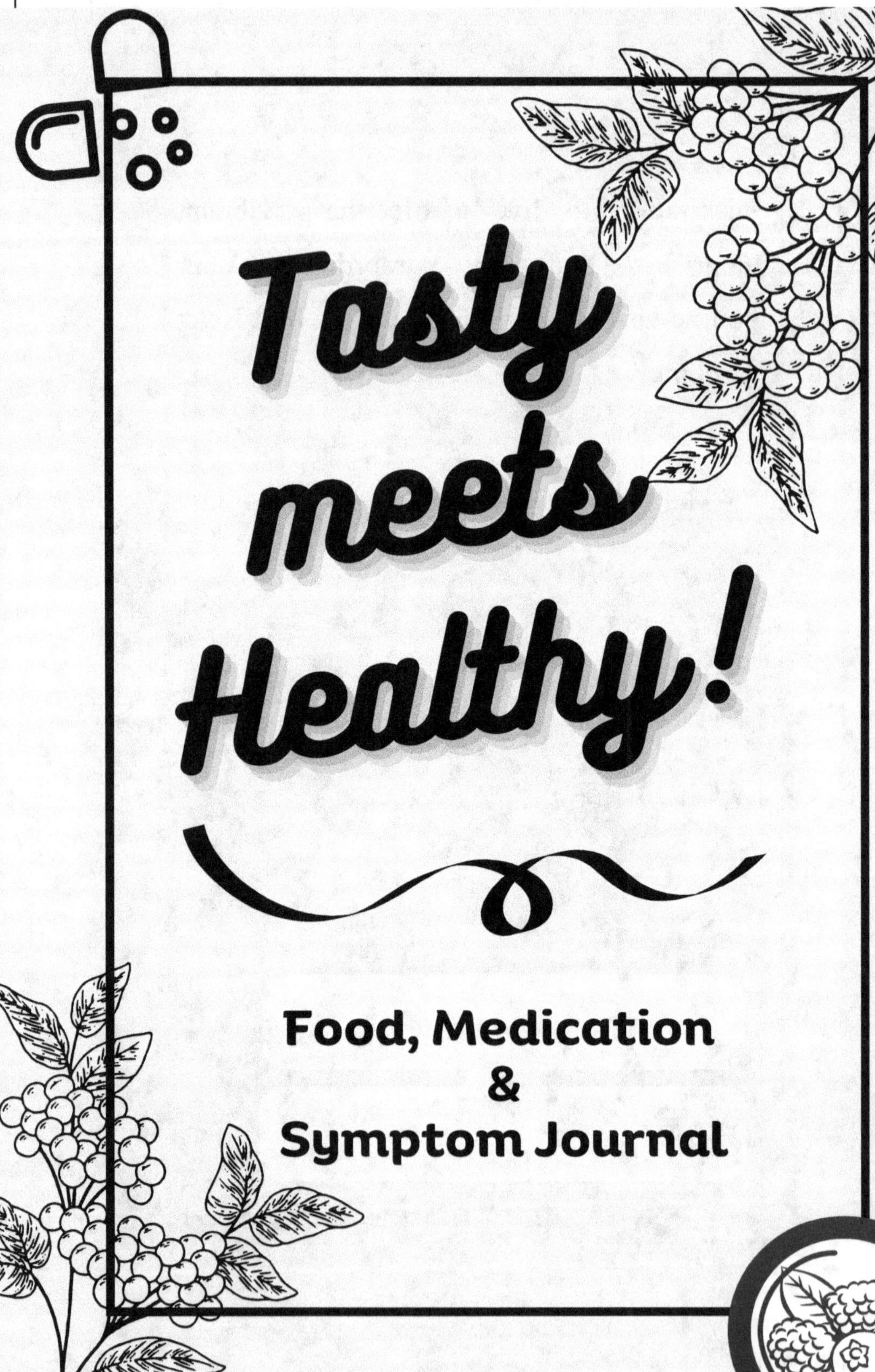

Tasty meets Healthy!

Food, Medication & Symptom Journal

FOOD, MEDICATION & SYMPTOM JOURNAL

Date: ______________________

Breakfast, Lunch, Dinner

- ___________________________________
- ___________________________________
- ___________________________________

Symptoms

- __________________ ○ ___________________
- ______________ ○ _______________

Medications

- ___________________________________
- ___________________________________
- ___________________________________

FOOD, MEDICATION
&
SYMPTOM JOURNAL

Date: ___________________

Breakfast, Lunch, Dinner

- _______________________________
- _______________________________
- _______________________________

Symptoms

- _______________ - _______________
- _______________ - _______________

Medications

- _______________________________
- _______________________________
- _______________________________

FOOD, MEDICATION
&
SYMPTOM JOURNAL

Date: _______________

Breakfast, Lunch, Dinner

- _________________________________
- _________________________________
- _________________________________

Symptoms

- _________________ - _________________
- _________________ - _________________

Medications

- _________________________________
- _________________________________
- _________________________________

FOOD, MEDICATION & SYMPTOM JOURNAL

Date: ______________

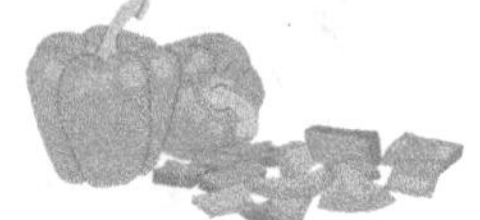

Breakfast, Lunch, Dinner

- ____
- ____
- ____

Symptoms

- ____
- ____

Medications

- ____
- ____
- ____

FOOD, MEDICATION & SYMPTOM JOURNAL

Date: ________________

Breakfast, Lunch, Dinner

- ________________________________
- ________________________________
- ________________________________

Symptoms

- __________________ __________________
- __________________ __________________

Medications

- ________________________________
- ________________________________
- ________________________________

FOOD, MEDICATION & SYMPTOM JOURNAL

Date: ______________

Breakfast, Lunch, Dinner

- ________________________________
- ________________________________
- ________________________________

Symptoms

- ___________ ● ___________
- ___________ ● ___________

Medications

- ________________________________
- ________________________________
- ________________________________

FOOD, MEDICATION
&
SYMPTOM JOURNAL

Date: ___________

Breakfast, Lunch, Dinner

- ___________________________________
- ___________________________________
- ___________________________________

Symptoms

- ___________________ ● ___________________
- ___________________ ● ___________________

Medications

- ___________________________________
- ___________________________________
- ___________________________________

FOOD, MEDICATION
&
SYMPTOM JOURNAL

Date: ______________

Breakfast, Lunch, Dinner

- ____
- ____
- ____

Symptoms

- ____________________   - ____________________
- ____________________   - ____________________

Medications

- ____
- ____
- ____

FOOD, MEDICATION & SYMPTOM JOURNAL

Date: _______________

Breakfast, Lunch, Dinner

- _______________________________________
- _______________________________________
- _______________________________________

Symptoms

- _____________ ● ___________________
- _____________   ● ___________________

Medications

- _______________________________________
- _______________________________________
- _______________________________________

FOOD, MEDICATION
&
SYMPTOM JOURNAL

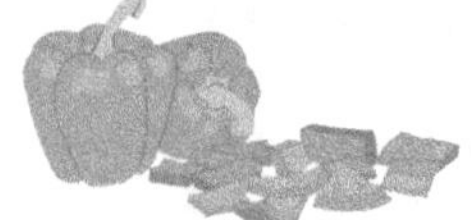

Date: ___________

Breakfast, Lunch, Dinner

- ______________________________
- ______________________________
- ______________________________

Symptoms

- ______________________________
- ______________________________

Medications

- ______________________________
- ______________________________
- ______________________________

FOOD, MEDICATION
&
SYMPTOM JOURNAL

Date: ___________________

Breakfast, Lunch, Dinner

- _______________________________
- _______________________________
- _______________________________

Symptoms

- _______________________________
- _______________________________

Medications

- _______________________________
- _______________________________
- 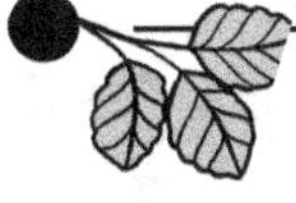 _______________________________

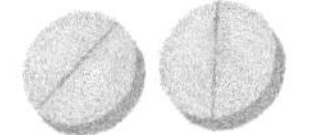

FOOD, MEDICATION
&
SYMPTOM JOURNAL

Date: ______________________

Breakfast, Lunch, Dinner

- _______________________________________
- _______________________________________
- _______________________________________

Symptoms

- ____________________ ● ____________________
- ____________________ ● ____________________

Medications

- _______________________________________
- _______________________________________
- _______________________________________

FOOD, MEDICATION & SYMPTOM JOURNAL

Date: ______________

Breakfast, Lunch, Dinner

- ____
- ____
- ____

Symptoms

- ___________________________ ● ______________
- ___________________ ● ______________

Medications

- ____
- ____
- ____

FOOD, MEDICATION
&
SYMPTOM JOURNAL

Date: ___________________

Breakfast, Lunch, Dinner

- ____
- ____
- ____

Symptoms

- _______________________ ● _______________________
- _______________________ ● _______________________

Medications

- ____
- ____
- ____

www.ingramcontent.com/pod-product-compliance
Lightning Source LLC
Chambersburg PA
CBHW070821260726
48660CB00005B/1944